Yaneisy Domínguez González
Yanelis Pérez Triana
Migdalia Reyes Ledon

Acute Myeloid Leukemia

Yaneisy Domínguez González
Yanelis Pérez Triana
Migdalia Reyes Ledon

Acute Myeloid Leukemia

Patients in the remission induction stage

ScienciaScripts

Imprint

Any brand names and product names mentioned in this book are subject to trademark, brand or patent protection and are trademarks or registered trademarks of their respective holders. The use of brand names, product names, common names, trade names, product descriptions etc. even without a particular marking in this work is in no way to be construed to mean that such names may be regarded as unrestricted in respect of trademark and brand protection legislation and could thus be used by anyone.

Cover image: www.ingimage.com

This book is a translation from the original published under ISBN 978-620-2-14333-2.

Publisher:
Sciencia Scripts
is a trademark of
Dodo Books Indian Ocean Ltd. and OmniScriptum S.R.L publishing group

120 High Road, East Finchley, London, N2 9ED, United Kingdom
Str. Armeneasca 28/1, office 1, Chisinau MD-2012, Republic of Moldova, Europe
Printed at: see last page
ISBN: 978-620-7-30288-8

SUMMARY:

Acute myeloblastic leukemias (AML) constitute between 15% and 20% of leukemias in pediatric patients. With the aim of describing patients diagnosed with acute myeloid leukemia in the remission induction stage, a descriptive, cross-sectional study was carried out in patients diagnosed with acute myeloid leukemia at the University Pediatric Hospital "José Luis Miranda" of Santa Clara. The study population consisted of 24 patients, who constituted the sample. The pediatric patients with Acute Myeloid Leukemia treated in the University Pediatric Teaching Hospital "José Luis Miranda", had a similar distribution according to sex, and with a higher frequency in the ages from 1 to 14 years old, mainly from Sancti Spiritus and Villa Clara, with predominance of white skin color, and normal weight nutritional status. Almost all of them presented anemia, leukocytosis and thrombocytopenia. The main complications were sepsis and febrile neutropenia, which showed no association with sex or age of the patients. Hyperleukocytosis was present in obese patients and cardiotoxicity predominated in overweight and obese patients. Slightly more than half of the patients died at the end of the study, and of these, one out of two died due to induction.

INDEX:

INTRODUCTION:

The first well-documented case of acute leukemia (AL) is attributed to Friedreich, but it was Epstein who used the term acute leukemie in 1889, and this led to the general recognition of the clinical distinctions between acute myeloid leukemia (AML) and chronic myelogenous leukemia. In 1878, Neumann, who proposed that the marrow was the site of blood cell production, suggested that leukemia originated in this organ, and used the term myelogenous leukemia. The availability of polychromatic stains as sequenced by Ehrlich's work, the description of the myeloblast and myelocyte by Naegeli, and the first recognition of the common origin of red blood cells and leukocytes by Hirshfiel laid the foundation for the current understanding of the disease.[1]

Cancer is the second leading cause of death in the world; the number of deaths is close to five million. There are around 14 million people affected by these proliferative processes, in addition to the economic and health consequences.[2]

Cancer is currently the second leading cause of death also in childhood, second only to accidents. The annual incidence of childhood cancer is estimated to be between 100 and 180 cases per million children. Leukemias account for 33% of all cancers occurring in infants, and rank first in all geographic areas, followed by lymphomas and tumors of the central nervous system.[2-6]

The annual incidence of all leukemias is 8 to 10 cases per 100,000 population. Among these hematological pathologies, acute leukemias (AL) represent a major health problem. [5,6]

The LA are a heterogeneous group of conditions involving disordered proliferation of a clone of hematopoietic cells. The absence of control mechanisms over cell differentiation is primarily due to changes in regulatory genes, leading to overproduction of cells unable to mature and function normally.[7-10]

Within ALL, lymphoblastic leukemias (ALL) account for 75% of cases. The prognosis of children with ALL has improved substantially over the last four decades. At the present time the probability of prolonged remissions or cure has increased from 5% in 1950, to 5-year survival rates of 86%,[8,9] however, childhood myeloid leukemias continue to represent a spectrum of hematopoietic malignancies with a difficult prognosis, especially considering that more than 90% of myeloid leukemias are acute.[1,4]

Acute myeloblastic leukemia (AML) is a neoplastic disease resulting from an uncontrolled clonal proliferation of abnormal precursor cells of myeloid, erythroid, monocytic, megakaryoblastic and less frequently mastocytic, basophilic and dendritic lineage. It infiltrates the bone marrow, produces a variable degree of cytopenias, involves different organs and/or systems and causes death by hemorrhage and/or infection.[11,12]

Acute myeloblastic leukemias (AML) constitute between 15% and 20% of leukemias in pediatric patients. They consist of clonal proliferation of immature myeloid progenitor cells, which leads to invasion of the bone marrow and in some cases, the liver, spleen, lymph nodes, as well as other organs and tissues.[11-14]

Advances in molecular studies, more intensive treatments and improved supportive care have increased the survival rate of this disease.[7-11].

1.5 to 3 new cases of AML are reported per 100,000 population, and their frequency increases with age. Its mortality rate increases progressively from infancy to reach 20 per 100,000 persons in the ninth decade of life. With the exception of the first month of life, when it is more frequent than ALL, the ratio of AML: ALL is 1:4. Its incidence remains stable until 10 years of age, increases moderately during adolescence, becoming the most frequent form in adults. There are no differences in incidence by gender or race.[15-17] There is little difference in incidence between those of African or European origin at any age.[14] The M3 AML subtype is more prevalent in Latin countries, accounting for 24% of AMLs, compared to 15% in Anglo-Saxon countries.[15-17]

The causes of malignant transformation are not absolutely known, although environmental or genetic factors that favor it have been identified. Among the environmental factors that intervene as causal agents are: high-dose radiation, long-term exposure to benzene or its derivatives, and treatment with alkylating agents and other cytotoxic agents. Among the genetic factors, chronic myeloproliferative disorders and myelodysplastic syndromes can evolve into AML.[18] Patients with immunodeficiency syndromes or diseases with chromosomal abnormalities have a higher incidence in the development of the pathology.[13]

There is a high concordance rate of AML in identical twins. Some viruses can also cause leukemia; among them, it is possible to mention retroviruses such as HTLV-1 and HTLV-2.[11,12]

AMLs can be classified by a variety of ways including morphology, surface markers, cytogenetics and oncogene expression. The distinction between AML and ALL is very important as they differ substantially in prognostic and therapeutic aspects.[17,18]

The first more comprehensive morphologic and cytochemical classification system for AMLs was developed by the French-US-British

(FAB) Cooperative Group. This system classifies AMLs based on morphology and immunologic detection of lineage markers.[19,20] Between 50% and 60% of children with AML are classified according to M1, M2, M3, M6 or M7 subtypes; about 40% have M4 or M5 subtypes. The response to cytotoxic chemotherapy among children with the different subtypes of AML is relatively similar. FAB subtype M3 is an exception since approximately 70% to 80% of children with AML achieve remission and cure with cell differentiation inducers plus chemotherapy.[21,22]

In 2002, the World Health Organization (WHO) proposed a new classification system that incorporated diagnostic cytogenetic information, role of myelodysplasia and previous cytostatic treatment that correlates more reliably with outcomes.[23]

The presentation of AML is reflected in symptoms and signs that depend on the degree of infiltration of the leukemia in the bone marrow or extra-marrow. In addition to the symptoms and signs, the diagnosis of acute myeloid leukemia is based on the results of the medulogram and bone marrow biopsy which are usually hypercellular, with the presence of 20 to 100% blast cells.[24]

A series of factors have been described that influence the prognosis and evolution of the disease, among the most important are cytogenetic and molecular abnormalities such as t(8,21) and t(15,17) translocations, inv (16), 11q23 gene rearrangement, FLT3 receptor tyrosinkinase activating mutations, internal tandem duplication, which together with other classical variables such as age, sex, initial leukocyte count, initial infiltration of the central nervous system (CNS), existence of genetic disorders such as Down syndrome, previous history of myelodysplastic syndrome or previous history of myelodysplastic syndrome, sex, initial leukocyte count, initial central nervous system (CNS) infiltration, the existence of genetic disorders such as Down syndrome, a history of previous myelodysplastic syndrome or aplastic anemia, and response to treatment, contribute significantly to determining different risk groups for the therapeutic management and prognosis of the disease.[22-24]

From 1962 onwards, therapeutic regimens combining multiple drugs with different mechanisms of action began to be used, for the first time for curative purposes. In the 1980s the West-German group BFM (Berlin-Frankfurt-Münster) began to use much more aggressive and shorter duration therapeutic schemes and high pharmacological doses were introduced; since then therapeutic protocols have focused on the intensification of treatments with known drugs, rather than on the introduction of new drugs.[25]

In the last decade, although the results of AML treatment have improved, they continue to be modest, and in practice most patients succumb to a disease that recurs and progresses after an initial response, or that is refractory to chemotherapy from the outset. AMLs therefore remain a major therapeutic challenge in the field of hematological malignancies.[19-21]

The Latin American Group for the Treatment of Malignant Hemopathies (GLATHEM), to which Cuba has belonged since 1973, has elaborated protocols similar to those of the BFM group with good results, especially in the last two decades. The University Pediatric Hospital "José Luís Miranda" of Santa Clara, started the GLATHEM studies since its foundation in 1973 together with the Institute of Hematology and Immunology.[26-29]

The researches that have been carried out in the University Pediatric Hospital "José Luís Miranda", in the city of Santa Clara on AML are not numerous. The lack of data on the particularities of AML in the context could be detrimental to patient care and hinder medical conduct, which justifies the following scientific problem:

What are the characteristics of patients with acute myeloid leukemia in the remission induction stage seen at the "José Luís Miranda" Pediatric Hospital?

OBJECTIVES:

General:

To describe patients diagnosed with acute myeloid leukemia in the remission induction stage.

Specific:

1. Characterize the group of patients according to the variables epidemiological and laboratory variables.

2. Identify the most frequent complications that appear during the remission induction stage.

3. To determine the association between complications and the variables studied.

4. To identify the causes of death in induction and the current status of the patients at the conclusion of the investigation.

THEORETICAL FRAMEWORK:

The treatment of children with cancer is one of the most complex challenges in pediatric practice. It begins with the absolute requirement for a correct diagnosis (including subtyping), followed by an accurate and comprehensive disease staging process to determine prognosis and culminating in appropriate multidisciplinary and often multimodality treatment, and requires assiduous assessment of the potential for tumor recurrence and possible late adverse effects of the disease or treatments used for the disease. Throughout treatment, the child with cancer should benefit from the expertise of specialized health care professionals trained in working with critically ill children.[24]

Leukemias can be defined as a group of malignancies in which genetic disorders of a particular hematopoietic cell result in unregulated clonal proliferation of cells. The progeny of these cells show a growth advantage over normal cellular elements due to their higher proliferation rate and lower incidence of spontaneous apoptosis. The consequence is a disruption of normal marrow function and ultimately marrow failure. Clinical features, laboratory findings and response to treatment vary according to the type of leukemia.[24,25]

Acute myeloid leukemia (AML), also known as acute nonlymphocytic leukemia, is a myeloid cell neoplasm that is caused by clonal transformation and proliferation of immature progenitors that displace and inhibit the growth of normal hematopoiesis and accounts for 15% to 20% of leukemias in pediatric patients.[21-23]

Acquired chromosomal inversions or translocations have been identified in 65% of acute leukemias (AL). These structural rearrangements affect gene expression and alter the normal functioning of cell proliferation, differentiation and survival.[18,30]

The pathophysiology of AML occurs by transformation of a myeloid hematopoietic cell to malignancy and subsequent clonal expansion of cells with suppression of normal hematopoiesis. Investigation of clonal chromosome abnormalities has helped to understand the genetic basis of leukemia.[31]

According to the FAB, AMLs are classified into: [19, 20,26,29]

M0: Acute myeloblastic leukemia without differentiation.

M0 AML does not express myeloperoxidase (MPO) at light microscopic grade, but may show characteristic granules on electron microscopy. M0 AML can be defined by the expression of cluster determinant (CD) markers such as CD13, CD33 and CD117 (c-KIT) in the absence of lymphoid differentiation. The classification of M0 assumes that leukemic blasts do not show morphologic or histochemical features of AML or acute lymphoblastic leukemia (ALL).

M1: Acute myeloblastic leukemia with minimal differentiation.

MPO expression detected by immunohistochemistry or flow cytometry. Blasts constitute more than 90% of non-erythroid cells, are medium to large in size with a variable nucleus-to-cytoplasm ratio and an oval nucleus with one or more nucleoli. It presents <10% granulocytic component in maturation. The presence of Auer rods in the cytoplasm is variable.

M2: Acute myeloblastic leukemia with differentiation.

In this subtype of AML there is evidence of myeloid maturation with a mature granulocytic component (promyelocytes to polymorphonuclear) greater than 10% of the non-erythroid cells and a monocytic component of less than 20%. Blasts constitute between 30% and 89% of the non-erythroid cells. The presence of Auer rods is more frequent than in M1 and myeloblasts contain azurophilic granules and prominent nucleoli.

M3: Acute promyelocytic leukemia (APL) hypergranular type.

The cells in M3 are characterized by hypergranulation of the promyelocytes with abundant Auer rods, sometimes forming bundles or palisades. If the granulations do not obscure the outline of the nucleus, the nucleus is reniform or folded. The MPO is strongly positive.

M3v:LPA, microgranular variant.

The cytoplasm has a very fine granulation that is sometimes difficult to see with light microscopy.

M3 AML presents, at the cytogenetic level, a t-translocation (15; 17) that is observed in both the hypergranular and microgranular varieties. In this subtype of AML, the cell membrane has intense procoagulant activity and the granules have proteolytic activity, which induce a picture of disseminated intravascular coagulation and consumption coagulopathy. Patients have a high tendency to develop intracranial and pulmonary hemorrhages before and a f t e r initiation of treatment.

M4: Acute myelomonocytic leukemia (AMML).

In this subtype of AML, blasts constitute more than 30% of the non-erythroid cells and have features of acute myeloblastic leukemia (M2) and acute monocytic leukemia (M5). Between 20% and 80% of the non-erythroid cells must have monocytic features or there must be more than 5×10^9 /L monocytes in peripheral blood. Serum or urinary lysozyme levels should be more than three times the normal value. Patients with a bone marrow consistent with M2 AML and peripheral monocytosis or increased lysozyme levels should be categorized as M4.

M4E0: AMML with eosinophiliain this variant up to 30% of eosinophils with morphological and cytochemical alterations are detected.

M5: Acute monocytic leukemia (AML0A).

The percentage of non-erythroid cells with monocytic characteristics exceeds 80%.

M5a or monoblastic leukemia, 80% of the non-erythroid marrow cells are monoblasts.

 M5b. LM0A with differentiation. Monoblasts constitute less than 80% of the monocytic component.

M6: Acute erythroid leukemia or erythroleukemia.

More than 50% of the medullary nucleated cells are erythroblasts and at least 30% of the non-erythroid cells are blasts. If erythroblasts are observed, but less than 30% of the non-erythroid cells are blasts, a myelodysplastic syndrome should be considered.

M7: Acute megakaryocytic leukemia.

Malignant megakaryoblasts are heterogeneous, ranging from small round cells similar to M1 or L2 subtypes to large atypical megakaryocytes. Megakaryoblasts are myeloperoxidase and black sudan negative, and may be PAS positive. Immunophenotyping with monoclonal antibodies recognizing platelet antigens, or ultrastructural examination of platelet peroxidase activity must be available to give a diagnosis of M7. This subtype is associated with myelofibrosis or increased marrow reticulin, so it is often not possible to obtain a sample in the marrow aspirate. It is common in patients with Down syndrome and AML.[19,20,26-29]

The classification system proposed by WHO in 2002 classifies AMLs as follows: [23]

- AML with characteristic or recurrent anancytogenetic

abnormalities. AML with t (8; 21) (q22; q22); (AML1/ETO).

AML with inv16 (p13q22) or t (16; 16) (p13; q22); (CBFß/MYH11).

AML with t (15; 17) (q22; q12); (PML/RARα and variants). AML with t

(6:9) (DEK/KAN).

LMA with t (9:11) (MLL/MLL-T3). AML with t (1; 22).

- AML related to myelodysplasia.

- AML, therapy-related. AML in relation to alkylating drugs.

Topoisomerase II inhibitor-related AML.

- LMA without further specification.

Minimally differentiated acute myeloblastic leukemia (FAB classification

M0). Non-maturing acute myeloblastic leukemia (FAB classification M1).

Acute myeloblastic leukemia with maturation (FAB classification M2).

Acute myelomonocytic leukemia (FAB classification M4).

Acute monoblastic leukemia and acute monocytic leukemia (FAB

classifications M5a and M5b).

Acute erythroid leukemias (FAB classifications M6a and M6b). Acute

megakaryoblastic leukemia (FAB classification M7).

- AML/transient myeloproliferative disorder in Down syndrome.

Acute basophilic leukemia.

Acute panmyelosis with myelofibrosis.

- Myeloid sarcoma. AML with positive Li antigen. Hybrid AML.

In AML, structural and/or numerical chromosomal alterations are detected
in 55% of patients. The findings of the cytogenetic study at diagnosis
constitute, together with age, the most important prognostic factor that
determines the response to treatment and survival. [13]

Based on these findings, patients with AML are classified into three cytogenetic groups: favorable, intermediate and unfavorable. Advances in the knowledge of molecular genetics in the last 15 years have allowed the identification of more than 100 mutations and/or gene rearrangements, which reflect the heterogeneity of the disease, contribute to better establish the prognosis of AML and provide clues to identify molecular targets. The main molecular alterations are described below:[5,35-39]

- FLT3 gene mutations:

This is one of the most frequent mutations in AML2, and is also associated with progression from myelodysplastic syndrome to secondary AML and acute promyelocytic leukemia (APL). Somatic mutations resulting in constitutive activation of the FLT3 gene have been identified in two functional domains of the receptor: the juxtamembrane domain and the tyrosine kinase domain.

From a clinical point of view, these mutations are relevant because of their prognostic impact and because they are an attractive target for molecular therapy. Patients with FLT3-ITD have a high leukocyte count and a high proportion of blasts in bone marrow; in addition, they more frequently have novocompartmental AML compared to those with the FLT3 gene in the germline (FLT3-WT). Multiple studies have shown that the presence of FLT3-ITD in patients with CN-AML is associated with poor prognosis, with decreased overall survival (OS) due to increased risk of relapse (RR). The prognosis appears unfavorable, particularly in the absence of germline allele expression or when the FLT3-ITD: FLT3-WT ratio is increased. The prognosis of patients with TKD point mutations is controversial.[40]

- Mutations of the c-KIT gene:

Approximately 80% of patients with AML have blasts expressing c-KIT.

Mutations can be of 2 types, those located in the extracellular portion of exon 8 and activation loop mutations in codon 816 of exon 172. The overall frequency of these mutations in AML is low (6-8% and 2%, respectively).

In certain AML subgroups the proportion of c-KIT mutations is higher, 12 and 16% in AML patients with t(8;21) and between 22 and 13% in patients with inv(16)/t(16;16), respectively.

Morphologically, 70% of patients with c-KIT gene mutation are classified as M2 FAB. In AML with t (8; 21), the c-KIT gene mutation is associated with leukocytosis at diagnosis. The incidence of c-KIT does not differ significantly between *de* novo AML, AML secondary to MDS, and AML secondary to chemotherapy treatment.[37]

- Mutations of the RAS genes:

In AML, the frequency of RAS mutations is independent of age, sex, initial white blood cell count, WHO classification, de novo and secondary AML. AML subgroups with inv (16)/t (16; 16) or inv (3)/t (3; 3) have a high frequency of RAS mutations, between 35 and 27%, respectively, in contrast to the low frequency in APL. The coexistence of RAS and FLT3 gene mutations is rare (2%). This rarity is consistent with the cooperative model of leukemogenesis described above. Most studies have not demonstrated prognostic impact of RAS gene mutations on OS, disease-free survival (DFS) and RR, although it is believed that RAS gene mutations may represent a factor of progression. [40,41]

- Mutations of the CBF complex:

Cytogenetically, the CBF group is defined by the presence of t(8;21)(q22;q22) or inv(16)(p13q22)/ t(16;16)(p13;q22). Both subgroups account for 15% of AMLs, are considered favorable prognostic, with high rates of CR and prolonged OS.

Patients with t (8; 21) and inv (16)/t (16; 16) benefit from consolidation therapy with high-dose cytarabine. Some studies show superior OS in patients with inv (16)/t (16; 16), compared to those with t (8; 21).[26, 29]

- CEBPA gene mutations:

CEBPA mutations contribute to the blockade of myeloid progenitor maturation in AML. They are frequently associated with FAB types M1 and M2, and have been observed in 7-9% of AML cases. In patients with AML and t (8; 21) (q22; q22), which is associated with M2 morphology, the AML1-ETO fusion protein inhibits CEBPA expression to levels insufficient for neutrophil differentiation. [42]

These data and the finding that the differentiation block observed in *knockoutcebpa* mice *is* similar to the M2 phenotype support the hypothesis that the CEBPA mutation and t (8; 21) may have a common pathway in the pathogenesis of AML.

There are 2 types of mutations, N-terminal, which prevent full expression of the protein, and C-terminal, which result in poor DNA binding or inhibit dimerization ability. Some patients have a single mutation, while others have multiple mutations. CEBPA mutations have been associated with favorable OS and SLE, have been described in patients with intermediate prognosis cytogenetics, and have not been observed in prognostic leukemias. Favorable, i.e., CBF7 leukemias. Clinical data suggest favorable response to high-dose cytarabine chemotherapy, with OS similar to that obtained in CBF leukemias.[42]

- MLL gene mutations:

The MLL gene, located on chromosome 11q23, shows recurrent chromosomal aberrations in patients with acute leukemia. Thus, 15% of patients with acute leukemia, myeloid, lymphoid, *de novo* or secondary to treatment with topoisomerase II inhibitors have alterations in this gene. Its presence in some series is associated with short CR duration and short SLE.[43-45]

AML manifests with signs and symptoms related to ineffective hematopoiesis (infection, hemorrhage, and impaired oxygen-carrying capacity). Common signs and symptoms in ALL (either myeloblastic or lymphoblastic) are bone pain, tiredness, fatigue, shortness of breath, myalgias and bleeding gums. In AML, laboratory data include a complete blood count showing anemia, thrombocytopenia, leukocytosis or neutropenia. A coagulopathy resembling disseminated intravascular coagulopathy, manifested by low fibrinogen and elevated activated partial thromboplastin time. Myeloblasts with Auer rods, which are elongated pieces of chromatin, are seen on peripheral blood examination.[1,11,12,46]

The diagnosis of AML involves an assessment of physical status, blood count data, bone marrow aspirate and biopsy. Examination of marrow morphology allows us to calculate the percentage of blasts in the marrow space and morphological data that distinguish between lymphoid and myeloid blasts. Specific staining, immunophenotyping and cytogenetic analysis are performed to confirm the diagnosis.[11,12,14]

Cytogenetic analysis allows us to examine the chromosomes of leukemic cells for genetic abnormalities. Genetic lesions responsible for the aberrant growth form of the leukemic clone include chromosomal losses or gains, resulting in a hyperdiploid or hypodiploid; chromosomal translocations leading to the formation of transformed fusion genes or dysregulation of gene expression; and inactivation of tumor suppressor gene function.[12]

Effective contemporary pediatric protocols for AML achieve complete remission rates of 75% to 90%. Of those patients who do not go into remission, about half have refractory leukemia and the other half die from complications of the disease or its treatment. In order to achieve complete remission it is usually necessary to induce profound bone marrow aplasia (with the exception of APL subtype M_3). Induction chemotherapy causes severe myelosuppression, with significant morbidity and mortality due to infection or hemorrhage.[1,8,9,11]

The two most effective drugs used to achieve remission are ARA-C and an anthracycline. The induction treatment regimens most commonly used in pediatrics use cytarabine and an anthracycline in combination with other drugs such as etoposide or thioguanine. The BFM group has studied cytarabine and daunorubicin plus etoposide (ADE) given over 8 days. Daunorubicin is the most commonly used anthracycline in induction regimens in children with AML, although idarubicin has also been used. [21,23,25]

The intensity of induction treatment influences the overall outcome of therapy. Although the presence of central nervous system (CNS) leukemia at diagnosis is more common in childhood AML than in childhood ALL,the reduction in overall survival directly attributable to CNS involvement is now less common in childhood AML. This finding is perhaps related both to the higher doses of chemotherapy used in AML (which can cross the blood-brain barrier) and to the fact that spinal cord disease in AML has not yet been effectively brought under long-term control as it has been in ALL. Children with AML subtypes M_4 and M_5 have the highest incidence of CNS leukemia.[25, 29]

The ideal antineoplastic agent would be one whose mechanism of action involves the distinguishing characteristics between normal cells and tumor cells, which would allow the malignant process to be combated with minimal damage to normal tissue. In general, the cellular targets of most antineoplastic agents are enzymes or substrates related to DNA synthesis or function. Despite the attempts of the medical and pharmaceutical world to achieve the ideal agent, it has not been possible to counteract the effects of chemotherapeutic drugs on non-tumor cells, which makes them agents with great destructive capacity and great complications.[30,31]

The main characteristics of the drugs used in the induction treatment of patients affected by this pathology will be presented below, with emphasis on the adverse effects that may be reported, since they constitute the main object of study of this research.

- ◆ Cytosine arabinoside (Cytarabine):[47]

It is an analog of deoxycytidine whose triphosphorylated metabolite. The arac-CTP competes with CTP for incorporation into DNA. The incorporated residue is a potent inhibitor of DNA polymerase. arac-CMP also inhibits the synthesis of glycoproteins and surface phospholipids, thus altering the structure and function of the cell membrane, and is specific to the cell cycle desynthesis phase.

Its bioavailability is low, 78% is eliminated in the urine and it crosses the blood-brain barrier well.it can be used intravenously, intrathecally and subcutaneously.its main interactions are with Allopurinol, colchicine, probenecid and sulfinpyrazone.

Its toxicity is shown at the level:

- Gastrointestinal: May manifest as abdominal pain, nausea, vomiting, stomatitis, diarrhea, pancreatitis and intestinal necrosis.

- Hematologic: may produce myelosuppression between 7 and 14 days.

- Dermatological: such as alopecia, rash, dermatitis, pruritus, urticaria.
- At the level of the central nervous system it can produce: chemical arachnoiditis, transient paraplegia, peripheral neuropathy, irreversible

leukoencephalopathy with nystagmus, ataxia, dysarthria, dysmetria, hallucinations. Convulsions, coma and death may also occur. It is mainly observed in relation to intrathecal overdose of the drug and appears in all its splendor between 7 and 8 days after drug administration.

- Renal: manifested by water retention and renal dysfunction.

- Hepatic: manifested by hepatic sinusoidal obstruction syndrome in dose cans, cholestasisintrahepatic and hepatic dysfunction.

- Others: Other manifestations of toxicity may also occur, such as: chemical keratoconjunctivitis in high doses, type I anaphylactoid reaction, cytosar syndrome characterized by fever, myalgias, altralgias, rashmaculopapular, asthenia and conjunctivitis, generally appearing between 6 and 12 hours after administration of the drug and should be treated with steroids, tachyarrhythmias and pneumonitis.[47-49]

  ♦ Anthracyclines:

They are a group of antitumor antibiotics that were described for the first time in 1963, extracted from Streptomyces Peucetius. Their first compound described was daunorubicin and later, through mutation induction, doxorubicin was obtained, which differs from its similar by a hydroxyl group that allows it to have a much broader antitumor pattern. The second generation of anthracyclines, including idarubicin and epirubicin, are of synthetic characteristics.

These compounds consist of several rings: a, b, c, d, which form a flat tetracyclic ring with variable side chains including doaunoxamine. Rings b and c possess quinone and hydroquinone which are responsible for the fluorescence of these products, the ability to form free radicals and to create metal ions. The planar structure of anthracyclines allows their interposition between DNA bases leading to topological changes resulting in inhibition of DNA, RNA and protein synthesis.

They are also compounds that inhibit topoisomerase II, which is the enzyme in charge of DNA chromosomal condensation; this inhibition results in the formation of DNA-enzyme-ANT complexes, producing DNA breaks. Another mechanism invoked in its action includes the generation of free radicals responsible for multiple tissue lesions. Free radicals actively participate in the pathogenic mechanism of the cardiotoxicity of these compounds. It has also been suggested that the interaction on intracellular signal transduction pathways could contribute to their antitumor action.[49,50]

Pharmacokinetics: Low availability by oral route, except for idarubicin which is well absorbed by this route, its use is exclusive for intravenous route, approximately 75% is bound to plasma proteins. In all cases anthracyclines present a hepatic metabolism where their different metabolites are formed, excretion is predominantly biliary and only epirubicin has a greater renal excretion as it forms soluble glucuronic derivatives.[51]

The compounds that can be found in this group are listed below:

o Daunorubicin: Presentation: 10mg/5ml and 20mg/10ml ampules.

o Daunorubicinaliposomal: Presentation: 50 mg ampoules that can only be diluted in 5% glucose solution, do not dilute in 0.9% physiological saline solution, a final concentration of 1 mg/ml should remain.

o Doxorubicin: Presentation: 10mg/5ml and 50mg/10ml ampules.

o Doxorubicinaliposomalpegilada:Presentation: 20 mg / 10 ml ampules, can only be diluted in glucose solution, do not use saline solution.

o Presentation: ampules of 5mg/5ml, 10mg/10ml and capsules of 5 and

25 mg.

- ○ Mitoxantrone: Presentation. 20 and 30 mg ampoules.[1,11,13]

Interactions: anthracyclines can sensitize normal tissues to the effect of radiotherapy and can give rise to recall reactions in areas that were irradiated. They should not be administered concomitantly with Allopurinol, colchicine, or probenecid since they increase uric acid levels in blood. Daunorubicin is incompatible with heparin, dexamethasone sodium and compounds containing aluminum.[1,11,13]

Toxicity:

- Intestinal gastrointestinal: anorexia, diarrhea, mucositis, stomatitis.

- Hematologic: myelosuppression.

- Dermatological: facial reddening, hyperpigmentation of the skin, rash, phlebosclerosis, in the case of mitoxantrone, blue coloration of the nails can be seen after treatment.

- Others: amenorrhea, hot flashes, oligospermia, azoospermia, chills, photosensitivity, amphylactoid reaction, elevated liver enzymes, red coloration of urine.

The most feared side effect with the use of anthracyclines is related to cardiotoxicity. Anthracyclines have been part of many therapeutic schemes used in patients with neoplastic diseases for more than three decades, and have been an important pillar in the achievements reached in terms of survival, mainly in pediatric age, If we take into consideration that acute lymphoid leukemia is the most frequent malignant hematological disease in children and that this therapeutic line is vital to achieve the cure of the disease, we can understand why multicenter studies are carried out for the follow-up and evolution of late complications of antineoplastic agents. Late effects on the cardiovascular system are among the most feared. [51,52]

There are different types of anthracycline cardiotoxicity depending, fundamentally, on the temporal sequence in which the manifestations appear and the type that is present. They can be divided into:

Acute: they appear during the infusion or during the following hours, are transient and present with electrical disturbances. It is less frequent than chronic and is rare after a single dose.

Most frequent electrical disturbances in this form:

- Non-specific alterations of the ST-T segment.

- Decreased QRS.

- QT segment prolongation.

- Sinus tachycardia.

- Supreventricular and ventricular arrhythmias.

- Conduction disorders (AV and bundle branch block).

Subacute: they occur days or weeks later, the most frequently described are pericarditis, myocarditis and congestive heart failure.

Chronic: we can observe clinically progressive chronicity of early onset, which is the most frequent and appears in the first year of treatment, characterized by cardiomyopathy and acute heart failure; clinically progressive chronicity of late onset can be seen up to 20 years after the end of treatment and is mainly characterized by heart failure, arrhythmias and ventricular dysfunction. The chronic form is the most frequent form of anthracycline cardiotoxicity and is generally related to the cumulative effect of the drug. [51-53]

The mechanism of toxicity may be due to the inhibition of the function of Topoisomerase II, which is a very important enzyme involved in the repair of DNA chains; these drugs also generate a large amount of free radicals from the iron-anthracycline complexes that can cause damage to the cytoplasmic membrane by lipid peroxidation, This seems to be the main cause of cardiotoxicity, since the heart has few enzyme complexes that limit free radical damage, which makes it very sensitive to oxidative stress.[9,54]

Myocardial damage is due to myocyte apoptosis, tissue injury and fibrosis. The effect of free radicals includes impaired calcium binding to the sarcoplasmic reticulum leading to calcium overload and contractility failure, defects in the expression of troponin, actin and myosin light chain genes, and the release of vasoactive amines and proinflammatory cytokines such as tumor necrosis factor and interleukin-2, but in addition, free radicals can activate intracellular signaling systems that trigger the programmed cell death machinery.[55]

Severe loss of myofibrils, mitochondrial disruption by the inflammatory process and nuclear degeneration have been observed as histopathological consequences of the changes described above. The degree of these changes has been used to define the severity of the damage; however, serial endomyocardial biopsies are not usually used because of their invasiveness and poor predictive value. There are several noninvasive methods that can be used for this purpose, such as ultrasound at rest and during exercise to measure the shortening fraction and radionuclide angiography to measure the ejection fraction. The presence of altered diastolic and systolic function suggests myocardial damage before its clinical expression, however, they are not early indicators of cardiotoxicity.[54,55]

Histological damage is not homogeneous; it is often of a mottled type, circumscribed to a wall or a ventricle, and the sequence of histological damage begins with edema of the sarcoplasmic reticulum, cytoplasmic vacuolization, myofibrillar degeneration, myocyte disruption, and fibrosis. Based on the severity of these changes, a classification of histological damage has been proposed.

Grade 0: No alterations.

Grade 1: Less than 5% of cells with early changes (loss of myofibrils and/or sarcoplasmic reticulum edema).

Grade 1.5: Between 5-15% of cells with definite changes (marked loss of myofibrils and/or cytoplasmic vacuolization).

Grade 2: Between 16-25% of cells with definite changes. Grade 2.5: 26-35% of cells with definite changes.

Grade 3: Diffuse cell damage greater than 35% with marked changes (loss of contractile elements, loss of intracellular organelles, mitochondrial and/or nuclear degeneration.[57,58]

The clinical course of anthracycline-induced left ventricular dysfunction is insidious, progressive and generally irreversible, although there may be spontaneous regression if the drug is discontinued at early stages of histological damage.[58]

Different techniques have been proposed for the evaluation of myocardial damage, the most widely used of which are as follows:

- Resting electrocardiography: it has been described that the analysis of heart rate variability could be an early index of cardiotoxicity, reflecting autonomic dysfunction with consensual systolic function.

- Radioisotopic ventriculography: it provides the left ventricular ejection fraction, which is altered before clinical signs of ventricular failure appear; it can be performed with a first-pass or topographic triggered technique (spect).

- Two-dimensional surface echocardiography: The calculation of left ventricular ejection fraction has an acceptable correlation with radioisotopic and angiographic studies. Its main disadvantage is its operator dependence and poor acoustic window. Being a method unrelated to ionizing radiation it has been preferred for use in the pediatric population. It is of interest to note that the evaluation of diastolic function with ultrasound by M-mode study of aortic root and mitral valve motility as well as other ECHO-Doppler parameters have been reported as early indicators of myocardial damage.

- Endomyocardial biopsy: Even though it is the reference technique it is a procedure that requires operators trained in its interpretation, in addition to its high cost and invasiveness, so its use has been left for those cases in which noninvasive studies are inconclusive.

- Indium-111-labeled antimyosin antibodies: although they appear to have very good sensitivity, their high cost and restricted availability limit their use for the study of chronic anthracycline cardiotoxicity.

- Quantification of adrenergic receptors with Iodine 123-labeled meta-iodobenzyl-guanidine.

- Plasma biochemical markers: endothelin-1, toponin T and natriuretic peptide B are the main markers.[57-59]

A series of factors have been established that predispose to or aggravate cardiovascular damage produced by these antineoplastic agents, which serve as a basis for specialists to prevent those patients who may develop greater damage.

Cardiotoxicity risk factors: [51,58]

- Age (extreme ages such as under 15 and over 65).

- Cumulative effect of the drug.

- History of previous heart disease.

- Use of radiotherapy from mediastinum o concomitance withother cardiotoxic drugs.

- Female sex.

- Vitamin E deficiency.

- Type of anthracycline used.

Mortality from this cause is considered to be very high, with lower survival in patients with dilated cardiomyopathy. Numerous strategies have been implemented to prevent these complications, mainly dose modifications, use of new anthracycline preparations, use of anticalcic drugs, beta-blockers, use of cardioprotectors such as iron chelating agents and free radical scavengers. The most commonly used drugs include dexrazoxane, amifostine, glutathione, vitamin E, erythropoietin, captopril, verapamil, probucol and melotonin. The most widely used is dexrazoxane. [57-60]

The definition of the maximum foreseeable dose for each anthracycline agent, together with the serial and non-invasive evolution of left ventricular function, is today the fundamental basis for the prevention of cardiotoxicity. [58]

Currently, the recommended dose caps for the use of anthracyclines are as follows: [56-60]

- Doxorubicin: >550 mg/m^2 sc (total dose).

- Daunorubicin: >550 mg/m^2 sc (total dose).

- Mitoxantrone: 100-200mg/m^2 sc (total dose).

- Epirubicin: 800 mg/m^2 sc (total dose).

- Idarrubicin: 120mg/m^2 sc(total dose)

Epipodophyllotoxins: In the 1950s, two compounds were developed from podoxyphyllin, known as ethopoxide and tenipoxide, which were approved by the FDA for the treatment of various malignancies in 1983. podoxyphyllin is an extract of Podopyillum pertatum and its antineoplastic properties were first described in 1946 although, prior to that time, it was used in the treatment of several other minor conditions.[61]

Etopoxide (VP-16): Its activity is mainly based on the cross-links it induces between DNA and proteins forming non-functional complexes and on the breaks it creates in the DNA strands, inducing an irreversible block to cells in pre-mitotic phases of the cell cycle by cancelling them in the synthesis phase or in G2, producing reversible inhibition of Topoisomerase II and allowing the DNA to carry out its replication and transcription functions.[61]

Its main route of administration is intravenous, although it can be administered orally. It is 90-95% bound to plasma proteins and its metabolism is hepatic and its conjugated metabolites do not have antineoplastic activity. It is important to note that patients with hypoalbuminemia will have greater toxicity at the same dose of the drug since the concentration of the free or protein-bound drug has a proportional relationship with the concentration of albumin. It does not cross the blood-brain barrier.[61,62]

Interactions: Different compounds have been described to increase the toxicity of ethopoxide among them the most mentioned are cisplatin, cyclosporine, and grapefruit juice.In turn this agent increases the anticoagulant effect of warfarin.

Toxicity:[63,64]

- Gastrointestinal: nausea, vomiting, anorexia, mucositis, constipation, abdominal pain, diarrhea, taste alterations, dysphagia.

- Hematologic: myelosuppression.

- Hepatic: hepatic dysfunction.

- Dermatological: phlebitis, epidermal toxic necrolysis, alopecia, hyperpigmentation, pruritus, dermitis.

- CNS: peripheral neurotoxicity.

- Others: hypersensitivity reactions, cardiotoxicity at high doses, Stevens-Johnson syndrome, second malignancies, transient hypotension that may be severe if administered in less than 30 minutes.

One of the major challenges in the treatment of AML is prolonging the duration of initial remission with additional chemotherapy or HSCT. In practice, most patients are treated with intensive chemotherapy after remission is achieved, because only a small subset has a matched related donor. This treatment uses drugs that were used at induction and usually includes high doses of ARA-C. [1]

Bone marrow transplantation in first remission has been evaluated since the late 1970s. Recent trials of transplantation in children with AML indicate that more than 60% to 70% of children who have matched donors available and who undergo allogeneic bone marrow transplantation during their first remission experience long-term remissions. Trials of allogeneic transplantation compared to chemotherapy or autologous transplantation have demonstrated superior outcomes in patients who were assigned to allogeneic transplantation based on the availability of a 6/6 or 5/6 related donor.[65-67]

Two approaches have emerged for the use of allogeneic bone marrow transplantation in first remission. In the first, patients who have favorable prognostic features at diagnosis only undergo transplantation after relapse the BFM group employs a combination of marrow response at day 15 (<5% blasts), and FAB subtype (M1 and M2 with Auer's rods, M3 or M4 E0) to define a good risk group.[44] Similarly, the UK Medical Research Council (MRC) has identified a good-risk group of patients with a 7-year survival after a complete remission of 78% and a disease-free survival of 59%. Patients in this group include those with t (8; 21), t (15; 17), FAB M3, inv16. This most likely identifies an equivalent group of patients included in the standard BFM risk group. The second approach is to offer allogenic bone marrow transplantation to all patients who have a matched related donor.[65-68]

With the passage of time, the arrival of new knowledge and technological advances that allow us to identify more specific molecular targets, the treatment of AML can be better stratified according to risk and the drugs to be used can have a greater antitumor effect and far fewer complications, which will allow a greater overall survival of our children and a better quality of life.

METHODOLOGICAL DESIGN:

A cross-sectional descriptive study was carried out with the purpose of describing patients diagnosed with acute myeloid leukemia in the referral induction stage at the University Pediatric Hospital "José Luís Miranda" of Santa Clara.

The study population consisted of 24 children diagnosed with acute myeloid leukemia in the remission induction stage. It was not necessary to apply sampling techniques.

VARIABLES:

VARIABLES	DESCRIPTION	MEASURING SCALE
Age.	Age in years completed.	❖ < 1 year ❖ 1 - 4 years ❖ 5 - 9 years ❖ 10 - 14 years ❖ 15 - 19 years
Sex.	According to biological sex.	❖ Male. ❖ Female.
Provenance.	Determine by provinces according to the political-administrative division and the area where the patient comes from.	❖ Santi Spiritus ❖ Villa Clara ❖ Ciego de Avila ❖ Cienfuegos ❖ Granma ❖ Matanzas
Skin color	According to skin color	❖ White ❖ Non-white
Nutritional status.	The child's nutritional status according to national tables will be taken into account.	❖ Malnourished. ❖ Delgado. ❖ Normal weight. ❖ Overweight. ❖ obese.
Hemoglobin	Debut value expressed in g/L	< 11 g/dl (anemia) 11 to 15 gr/dl (normal)
Leukocytes	Debut value expressed x 10 /L^9	< $5*10^9$ /L (leukopenia) 5 to 11 $*10^9$ /L (normal) > $11*10^9$ /L (leukocytosis)
Platelets	Debut value expressed x	< $150*10^9$ * L

	10 /L.^{9}	(Thrombocytopenia) from 150 to 450 $*10^9 * L$ (normal)
Complications	Events occurring in the remission induction stage that affect the patient's evolution and prognosis.	Sepsis. Febrile neutropenia. Hemorrhage before chemotherapy. Lysistumoral syndrome. Hemorrhage due to chemotherapy. Cardiotoxicity. Hyperleukosis.
Causes of death in the induction stage.	Events that caused the death of the patient during the remission induction stage (direct causes of death).	Severe sepsis Intraparenchymal hemorrhage to +CID Intraparenchymal hemorrhage to +SDMO Intraparenchymal hemorrhage.
Current status	Survival status of the patient at the time that the research culminates.	Vivo Died in induction Died from other cause

Techniques and procedures:

The source to be used was the clinical history of each patient, from which all the variables reflected in the study were obtained.

Information processing:

The data collected from the clinical history were entered into a data file in SPSS, version 15.0, and with the help of this statistical package, data and graphs were created in order to establish relationships between the variables.

Frequency distribution tables were created with absolute (number of cases) and relative (per hundred) values.

From the inferential point of view, the Chi-square test was applied to determine whether there is statistical independence between the variables (when p>0.05) or not, in the case of a contingency table with expected values less than 5.

Ethical considerations:

The study was conducted in accordance with the provisions of the declaration of the World Helsinki Assembly, after consultation with the review and approval by the Institutional Scientific Committee and the Research Ethics Committee. Only information from the clinical records was collected, with no interventions on the patients. The confidentiality of the information was maintained and the identity of those included in the study was not published.

RESULTS:

The distribution of children with acute myeloid leukemia by age and sex is shown in **Table 1.**

Of the male sex, 12 patients were identified, which constituted 50 %, and of the female sex, 12 patients constituted the remaining 50 %.

According to age, the distribution was similar in the groups of 1 to 4 years, 5 to 9 years, and 10 to 14 years, with 6 children in each of these groups, representing 25% respectively. Below 1 year of age and between 15 and 19 years, 3 cases were found in each group, representing 12.50 % respectively.

The significance, p = 0.406 of the Chi-square statistic, corroborates that the distribution by age group was similar in males and females, with no significant differences between them.

The place of residence of the patients (Table 2) shows that 10 cases (41.67 %) were from Sancti Spiritus province. In second place were 6 patients from Villa Clara, which represented 25% of the total. From other provinces, Ciego de Avila and Cienfuegos with 3 patients from each province (12.50 %) respectively, Granma and Matanzas with 1 patient from each (4.17 %) respectively.

Skin color (Table 3) white was the characteristic of 21 patients comprising 87.5 % of the sample. Only 3 patients were non-white for a
12.5 %.

The nutritional status of the pediatric patients with Acute Myeloid Leukemia (table 4 and graph 1), shows that 18 children who constituted 75 % were normal weight. They were followed in frequency by those with a weight above normal values with 1 overweight (4.17 %) and 3 obese (12.50 %).Only 2 patients (8.33 %) were classified as thin according to their nutritional status.

The results of complementary tests at diagnosis are shown in Table 5.

Regarding hemoglobin, anemia was present at diagnosis in 23 patients, these constituted 95.83 % of the total studied.

At diagnosis, 18 children (75 %) presented leukocytosis and 4 patients (16.70 %) presented leukopenia. Only 2 cases (8.30 %) presented normal values of leukocytes.

Thrombocytopenia was manifested in 17 patients, which made up 70.80% of the total studied.

Table 6 and Graph 2 show the complications that occurred in pediatric patients with Acute Myeloid Leukemia; the table establishes the relationship of these complications with the sex of the children.

Sepsis was the main complication occurring in 22 patients and constituted 91.67 %, with a similar distribution in males and females, p = 0.460.

Febrile neutropenia was the second complication, occurring in 87.50 %, as it manifested in 21 children with AML. Its manifestation did not depend on gender, p
= 1.000.

Hemorrhage before chemotherapy was a complication that occurred in 15 patients (62.50 %), also with similar manifestation in both sexes, p = 0.202.

Tumor lysis syndrome was present in 10 cases (41.67 5). It occurred in 25 % of the male cases and in 58.33 % of the female cases, although they did not show significant differences, p = 0.214.

Hemorrhage due to chemotherapy was a complication presented in 6 patients (25 %), of these in 5 males and 1 female, although they were not significantly different (p = 0.157).

Cardiotoxicity, manifested in 8 patients (33.33 %), with equal frequency in males and females, p = 1.000.

Hyperleukocytosis was manifested in only 2 patients (8.33 %), both of whom were male.

Table 7 establishes the relationship between complications and patient age, showing that the occurrence of complications did not show significant differences in the age groups studied; in all cases, statistical significance was greater than 0.05.

Table 8 shows the relationship between the complications presented by patients with acute myeloid leukemia in the remission induction stage and nutritional status, and shows that the presence of these complications did not depend on nutritional status, except for cardiotoxicity and hyperleukosis. Cardiotoxicity showed a significant association, p = 0.019. In this complication, its presence was observed in all overweight and obese patients. The two patients who presented hyperleukosis were obese, p = 0.002.

Table 9 shows the causes of death by sex in pediatric patients with acute myeloid leukemia in the remission induction stage. A total of 7 deaths occurred with a lethality of 29.17 % of the patients. Of these, 6 were female with a lethality of 50 % in this sex and only 1 male, with a lethality of 8.33 % in males, mortality depended significantly on sex, being higher in females, p = 0.0247.

According to the causes, there were 3 deaths due to severe sepsis (12.50 %, 1 due to intraparenchymal hemorrhage +CID (4.17 %), 1 due to intraparenchymal hemorrhage +SDMO (4.17 %), and 2 due to intraparenchymal hemorrhage (8.33 %), of which one was female and one male.

The current status of the pediatric patients with acute myeloid leukemia (Table 10) shows that 11 cases are alive, representing 45.83% of the sample, 29.17% (7 cases) died due to induction and 6 patients (25%) died due to other causes.

DISCUSSION OF THE RESULTS:

Cancer in children and adolescents is very rare worldwide. It is estimated that its incidence fluctuates between 1.5 and 2% of all malignant neoplasms detected each year. In Cuba, an annual average of 300 new cases are diagnosed in children, a figure that fluctuates annually.[9,10,28]

In the present study we observed that the distribution by sex was equal with 50 percent in each sex and that the distribution by age had the same frequency from one to 14 years, with fewer patients under one year and over 15 years.

When consulting the bibliography in a descriptive Cuban study on the clinical and epidemiological characteristics of leukemias in children, carried out in the Hematology Service of the Hospital Infantil Sur Docente de Santiago de Cuba,[10] found a predominance of the disease in the age group over 8 years old and in males.

Ducasse K, et al,[46] in patients with acute myeloid leukemia found a median age of 9 years with a male predominance of 63%.

Menéndez Veitía A and collaborators,[62] in a study of the treatment of acute myeloid leukemia in children in Cuba, of a total of 46 patients included, found a predominance of the male sex (n = 32) with a median age of 9 years.

Peña JA and collaborators,[8] determined that pediatric leukemias occurred in ages 7 to 15 years with 53.8% in children and adolescents, and with age peaks at 5 and 9 years with 15.4% and 9.6% respectively and median of 7.8 ± 4.0 years. The incidence of AML was higher in female sex (60%) with a female to male ratio of 1.5:1. This author found a similar distribution of cases from 1 to 14 years without significant differences.

In the casuistry studied, the patients resided fundamentally in the provinces of Sancti Spiritus and Villa Clara, it would be convenient in future investigations to carry out spatiotemporal distributions of Acute Myeloid Leukemia in the pediatric age, to determine the municipalities of origin of these to establish possible spatial associations of the cases. In this regard, in the literature there is a study that establishes a comparison between the risk period of childhood leukemia of cases diagnosed in the United States in different areas, in the north (above 40° latitude), such as Seattle, Nebraska, Lowa, Detroit and Connecticut with cases diagnosed in the southern United States (less than 40° latitude), including San Francisco, Utah, New Mexico and Atlanta and found more complex trimodal patterns, with seasonal peaks in April, August and December for the north, and seasonal peaks in February, July and October for southern localities. The authors suggest that these peaks may coincide with seasonal elevations in the occurrence of allergies and infectious processes, elements that are capable of promoting lymphocytic proliferation.[69]

In the patients studied, white skin color predominated in 21 cases that constituted 87.5 % of the sample. We consider that it is not associated to the presence of the disease, but to the distribution of the ethnic characteristics of the Cuban population and of the central regions of the country, which had the highest frequency of cases.

Authors consulted,[15-17] refer to the fact that the incidence of leukemias in the pediatric age group does not show differences by sex or race. There are no references of studies showing these characteristics.

In the present study, an adequate nutritional status of children with Acute Myeloid Leukemia was evidenced, none was malnourished, and normopese children predominated, which speaks in favor of the quality of pediatric care provided in Cuba, governed by the mother and child program. The Cuban studies consulted show similar results with a higher frequency of normopese children at the time of diagnosis of the disease.[9,10,28,46]

The patients who made up the series studied at the time of diagnosis presented anemia, leukocytosis and thrombocytopenia, results that together with the clinical and other diagnostic means corroborate the presence of the disease.

González Gilart G,[10] in a Cuban study found that among the clinical forms of presentation, anemic syndrome, purpura-hemorrhagic manifestations and fever stood out.

Other authors such as Naoe T,[70] Hernández Cruz C and collaborators,[56] and Fernández HF,[57] show similar results of the complementary tests used for the diagnosis of the disease.

Regarding complications, in the present study sepsis, febrile neutropenia and hemorrhage before chemotherapy were observed in almost all the children, with similar distribution according to sex. Tumor lysis syndrome was more frequently observed in females and hemorrhage due to chemotherapy and hyperleukocytosis in males, but no statistically significant differences were found. Cardiotoxicity occurred with low frequency and similar distribution by sex.

We agree with what has been stated about complications in the induction stage in the literature consulted. It is referred that due to profound and prolonged neutropenia secondary to chemotherapy, bacterial and fungal infections are the major cause of morbimortality in patients with AML, which is reflected in prolonged periods of hospitalization, increased use of broad-spectrum antimicrobials, appearance of antimicrobial resistance and increase of associated superinfections.[71-73]

Ducasse K et al,[46] characterizes the episodes of febrile neutropenia in patients with AML in whom he observed a greater number of days of fever, higher frequency of arterial hypotension and sepsis and prolonged hospitalizations in acute care wards. The frequency of sepsis found by this author was 27.7% in the group with AML and he found infectious foci in 70% of these patients, the most frequent being: bacteremia (23%), respiratory (27%) and digestive (25%), mainly of bacterial etiology. This author concludes that episodes of febrile neutropenia in children with AML require a more aggressive diagnostic and therapeutic approach, related to their severity.

González Gilart G et al.,[10] determined that fever was the predominant symptom in all children with AML, and found purpuric-hemorrhagic manifestations in 76.6 % of them. They showed infections as the most frequent complication, which represented 95.7 %, followed by hemorrhages (90 %).

Cavagnaro S F,[74] regarding tumor lysis syndrome in pediatrics, refers that it is a metabolic emergency derived from the rapid and massive destruction of tumor cells spontaneously or secondary to cytolytic cancer therapy. This situation produces an enormous imbalance of the internal environment by releasing large amounts of intracellular contents into the interstitial and intravascular space, with serious and even fatal clinical consequences. Adequate recognition of the risk factors that can cause this syndrome, as well as its prevention and specific treatment have substantially reduced complications and improved the survival of these patients.

Regarding this complication other authors,[75-77] identify associated risk factors such as: large or extensive tumors (tumor >10 cm in diameter or leukocytosis > 50 000 x mm^3), extensive bone marrow involvement, tumors with high cell proliferation rate or those with high sensitivity to chemotherapeutic agents, and among the predisposing host factors: elevated serum lactate dehydrogenase levels (greater than twice the upper limit of normal), baseline hyperuricemia or hyperphosphatemia, pre-existing renal dysfunction, volume depletion and oliguria. There are no references in the literature of its association with epidemiological variables of the patients.

A frequent complication of acute myeloid leukemia is hyperleukocytosis. Its presentation has been associated with reduced survival. Its recognition can be difficult, since it can simulate the presence of infections and hemorrhagic complications associated with acute leukemia.[78] In the present study we found only two patients with this complication, they presented an unfavorable evolution with other associated complications and died although not in induction.

Peña JA,[8] reported the incidence of complications in 35 cases (67.3%) and the main complications were infectious in 23 patients (65.7%), of which 22.8% occurred in the induction phase. Tang et al,[79] in Japan in2009, found 27.2% of infectious complications in this stage.

Hemorrhagic complications were the third most frequent in the present study, with a higher percentage than that reported by Peña JA,[8] , who determined that hemorrhagic complications were the most frequent after infectious complications with 11.4%. Kim et al,[80] in Korea in 2006 found 18.9%.

It is referred by several authors,[8,53,81] that this type of complications is common in individuals with hematologic cancer, bleeding occurs for different reasons, among them, alteration in the function and number of platelets, deficiencies in coagulation factors, circulating anticoagulants and defects in vascular integrity. Hemorrhage has been considered a cause of premature death in children with leukemia. Potential associated risks include hyperleukocytosis, leukemia immunophenotype, especially acute promyelocytic leukemia, thrombocytopenia and infection-associated.

In the present study, cardiotoxicity was present in 33.33% of the patients. It is stated in the literature that anthracyclines, considered today as the most important antitumor drugs, have precisely this limitation; their clinical utility is restricted by the appearance of cardiomyopathies.[82,83]

The frequency of subclinical myocardial alterations reported after treatment with anthracyclines reaches up to 57% and of symptomatic cardiac alterations, up to 16%.[84]

It has been described that the highest frequency of cardiotoxicity is found with a cumulative dose higher than 450 mg/m^2 SC. However, it has been shown that myocardial damage already exists at lower doses.[82]

In the patients included in the study, the complications presented in the remission induction stage did not depend on the age of the patients; the distribution of these groups was similar.

Peña JA,[8] in the study cohort of his research found that 55.8% of the male sex presented complications, with infectious complications being the most frequent in 60.9%. Regarding age, this author found complications in 46.2% of the age group 0 to 6 years and the main complications were infectious in 60.9%. In the 7 to 15 years age group he found 64% of complications.

With respect to nutritional status in the casuistry studied, a relationship of complications such as cardiotoxicity and hyperleukocytosis was observed depending on nutritional status, predominantly in overweight and obese patients. With these results we cannot establish causal association, since it is a descriptive study with a small sample size, this distribution could be due to chance. There are no references in the literature on the influence of body weight on these complications.

In the patients studied, mortality during induction was 29.17 %, with dependence on sex, only one death was male and almost all were female. The main cause of death was severe sepsis. At the time of completing the investigation, 45.83 % were alive, since a quarter of the patients had also died of other causes not related to the induction to remission process.

It is stated in the literature that the five-year survival rate of the different types of leukemia has improved substantially in the last decades, thus, in the 60's a child with leukemia had a 5% chance of survival at five years; at the end of the 70's, 50% in ALL and rarely a child with AML survived. In the period 1990-2000 the survival rates of leukemias became similar when comparing the results of the USA, Europe and America.[9]

A study conducted in Chile,[46] shows that the five-year survival rate for AML in children under 15 years of age was 50%. Despite the chemotherapy treatment (QT) used, 30% of children experience relapse of the disease and 10% do not respond to QT.

Several authors,[54,61,62,85] suggest that the lower survival rate in patients with AML is due to toxic effects and morbidity and mortality associated with the aggressive QT regimens needed to try to cure this pathology.

The tendency to die more in the group of children with AML could be explained by the existence of other causes of mortality described in this group of patients, such as massive hemorrhages (specifically in M3 AML), hydroelectrolytic alterations, renal dysfunction and neurological compromise.[15-217,68,86]

González Gilart G, et al,[10] regarding mortality identified 66.6% of deaths in pediatric patients with acute myeloid leukemia in Santiago de Cuba from 2006 to 2010.

Peña JA,[8] calculates the relative risk (RR) of infectious and hemorrhagic complications and mortality. The risk of infectious complications and death was 2.06 (95% CI 0.26-16.65) and 1.93 (95% CI 0.28-13.32) for hemorrhagic complications, although the results were not statistically significant (p>0.05). Survival at 120 weeks was 60% for AML.

CONCLUSIONS:

Pediatric patients with Acute Myeloid Leukemia treated at the University Teaching Pediatric Hospital "José Luis Miranda" during the study period, had a similar distribution according to sex, and with greater frequency in the ages from 1 to 14 years, mainly from Sancti Spiritus and Villa Clara, with predominance of white skin color, and normal weight nutritional status. Almost all of them presented anemia, leukocytosis and thrombocytopenia. The main complications were sepsis and febrile neutropenia, which showed no association with sex or age of the patients. Hyperleukocytosis was present in obese patients and cardiotoxicity predominated in overweight and obese patients. Slightly more than half of the patients died at the end of the study, and of these, one out of two died due to induction.

BIBLIOGRAPHIC REFERENCES:

1. Lichtman MA, Liesveld JL. Acute myelogenous leukemia. In: Williams Hematology. 8th ed [Internet]. New York: McGraw-Hill; 2010. p.1056 - 69. Available from: http://accessmedicine.mhmedical.com/content.aspx?bookid=358§i onid=39 835911

2. Ferlay J, Shin HR, Bray F, Forman D, Mathers C, Parkin DM (2010) Estimates of worldwide burden of cancer in 2008: GLOBOCAN 2008. Int J Cancer [Internet]. 2010 [cited May 2014]; 127(12): [approx. 14 p.]. Available from: http://onlinelibrary.wiley.com/doi/10.1002/ijc.25516/pdf

3. Bosetti C. Childhood cancer mortality in Europe, 1970-2007. Eur J Cancer [Internet]. 2010 [cited May 2014]; 46(2): [approx. 10 p.]. Available from: http://www.ncbi.nlm.nih.gov/pubmed/19818600

4. Couto AC, Ferreira JD, Koifman RJ, Monteiro GT, Pombode-Oliveira MS, Koifman S. Trends in childhood leukemia mortality over a 25-year period. J Pediatr [Internet]. 2010 [cited May 2014]; 86(5): [approx. 5 p.]. Available from: http://www.scielo.br/pdf/jped/v86n5/en_v86n5a09.pdf.

5. Maloney K, Greffe BS, Foreman NK; Giller RH, Quinones RR, Gram. DK, et al. Acute Lymphoblastic Leukemia In: Levin M, Sondheimer J, Deterding R. Current diagnosis and treatment in pediatrics. 20th ed [Internet]. New York: McGraw-Hill; 2011. p. 853- 856. [Internet]https://www.fgq77.files.wordpress.com/2013/07/current_diag nosis_a nd_treatment_pediatrics.pdf

6. Guillerman RP, Voss SD, Parker BR. Leukemia and Lymphoma. Radiol Clin N Am [Internet]. 2011 [cited May 2014]; 49(4). [Internet]

www.radiologic.theclinics.com/article/S0033-8389(11)00062-5/pdf.

7. Riquelme S V, García B C. Imaging studies in the early diagnosis of leukemia in pediatrics. Rev. Chil. Radiol [Internet]. 2012 [cited May 2014]; 18(1): [approx. 5 p.]. Available at: http://www.scielo.cl/pdf/rchradiol/v18n1/art06.pdf

8. Peña JA, Pantoja JA, Acosta ÁM, Argotty-Pérez E, Mafla AC. Associated complications and survival analysis of children with acute leukemias treated with the BFM-95 protocol. Rev Univ Health [Internet]. 2014 [cited Jan 2015]; 16(1). Available from: http://www.scielo.org.co/scielo.php?script=sci_arttext&pid=S0124-71072014000100002.

9. Vera AM, Pardo C, Duarte MC, Suárez A. Analysis of pediatric acute leukemia mortality at the National Cancer Institute. Biomedica [Internet]. 2012 [cited May 2014]; 32: [approx. 5 p.].Available from: http://www.scielo.org.co/scielo.php?script=sci_pdf&pid=S0120-41572012000300006&lng=en&nrm=iso&tlng=en.

10. Gonzalez Gilart G, Salmon Gainza SL, Querol Betancourt N, et al. Clinical epidemiological characteristics of leukemias in children. MEDISAN [Internet]. 2011 [cited April 2015]; 15(12). Available en: http://scielo.sld.cu/scielo.php?script=sci_pdf&pid=S1029-30192011001200005&lng=es&nrm=iso&tlng=es

11. Creutzig U, Van den Heuvel-Eibrink MM, Gibson B, Dworzak MN, Adachi S, De Bont E, et al. Diagnosis and management of acute myeloid leukemia in children and adolescents: recommendations from an international expert panel. Blood [Internet]. 2012 [cited April 2015]; 120 (16). Available from:

http://www.ncbi.nlm.nih.gov/pubmed/22879540

12. Harrison CJHills RK, Hills RK, Moorman AV, Grimwade DJ, Hann I, Webb DK, et al. Cytogenetics of Childhood Acute Myeloid Leukemia: United Kingdom Medical Research Council Treatment Trials AML 10 and 12, J. Clin. Oncol [Internet]. Jun 2010 [cited April 2015]; 28. Available from: http://www.ncbi.nlm.nih.gov/pubmed/20439644.

13. Balgobind BVRaimondi SC, Harbott J, Zimmermann M, Alonzo TA, Auvrignon A, et al. Novel prognostic subgroups in childhood 11q23/MLL-rearranged acute myeloid leukemia: results of an international retrospective study. Blood [Internet]. Sep 2009 [cited April 2015]; 114(12). Available from: http://www.ncbi.nlm.nih.gov/pubmed/19528532

14. Niewerth DCreutzig U, Bierings MB, Kaspers GJ. A review on allogeneic stem cell transplantation for newly diagnosed pediatric acute myeloid leukemia. Blood [Internet]. Sep 2010 [cited 2015 Apr 2015]; 116. Available from: http://www.ncbi.nlm.nih.gov/pubmed/20538803.

15. Burnett A, Wetzler M, Löwenberg B. Therapeutic Advances in Acute Myeloid Leukemia. J Clin Oncol [Internet]. 2011 [cited March 2013]; 29(5). Available from: http://jco.ascopubs.org/content/early/2011/01/10/JCO.2010.30.1820.full.pdf

16. Dombret H. Optimal acute myeloid leukemia therapy in 2012. Educational Program EHA 2012; 6:41-48

17. Estey E. Annual Clinical Updates in Hematological Malignancies: A Continuing Medical Education Series: Acute myeloid leukemia: 2012

update on diagnosis, risk stratification and management. ASH Educational Material. ASH; 2011.

18. Alencar Á, Buessio R, Scheinberg P. Acute leukemias, In: Brazilian Manual of Clinical Oncology; [Internet]2013. Sao Pulo, Brazil: regional council of stadium medicine. Available at: https://mocbrasil.com/moc-hemato/neoplasias-malignas/9-leucemias-agudas-introducao.

19. Döhner H. Implication of the molecular characterization of acute myeloid leukemia. Hematology Am Soc Hematol Educ Program. [Internet] 2007[cited January 2015]. Available from: http://www.ncbi.nlm.nih.gov/pubmed/18024659

20. Gilliland G, Jordan CT, Felix CA. The molecular basis of leukemia. American Society of Hematology Education Program Book[Internet] 2007[cited January 2015]. Available from: http://www.ncbi.nlm.nih.gov/pubmed/15561678

21. Rubnitz JE. Childhood acute myeloid leukemia. Curr Treat Options Oncol, Feb[Internet] 2008[cited January 2015]; 9(1). Available from: http://www.cancer.gov/types/leukemia/patient/child-aml-treatment-pdq

22. Rubnitz JE et al. Acute mixed lineage leukemia in children: the experience of St. Jude Children's Research Hospital. Blood 2009; 113(21):5083-5089.

23. Rubnits JE, Gibson B, Smith FO. Acute Myeloid Leukemia. Pediatr Clin N Am [Internet]. 2008 [cited February 2013]; 55(1). Available from: http://www.elsevier.com/copyright.

24. David G. Tubergen, Archie Bleyer, Kim Ritchey. Acute myeloid leukemia. In: Nelson, A Treatise on Pediatrics. 19th ed. Philadelphia: Saunders Elservier; 2011.

25. NCCN. NCCN Clinical Practice Guidelines in Oncolgy. Acute

Myeloid Leukemia; [Internet] 2009 [cited 21 Feb 2013] Available from: http://www.nccn.org.

26. All Study Task Force. ALL IC-BFM 2007 13th Annual meeting of I-BFM-SG. Budapest Hungary; May 3-5, [Internet] 2007 [cited 12 Jan 2013] Available from: http://www.infomed.sld.cu

27. Garay G, Aversa LA, Svarch E, Sackman Muriel F, Drelichman G, Santareli MT. Progress in the treatment of acute lymphoid leukemia in children. GATLA/GLATHEM experience. Blood 1989; 34 (2): 136 - 43.

28. Vergara B, Svarch E. Childhood acute lymphoblastic leukemia. Post-completion of treatment follow-up in 430 patients. Rev Esp Pediatr 2004; 60: 348 - 54.

29. Svarch E, González A, Vergara B, Campos M, Dorticós E, Espinosa E, et al and Grupo para el Estudio y Tratamiento de las Hemopatías Malignas en Cuba (GETHMAC). Treatment of leukemias in Cuba 1973-1995. Rev Cubana Hematol Inmunol Hemoter 1996;12: 112 - 8.

30. Camañas Troyano C. Ponatinib: new alternative for the treatment of resistant chronic myeloid leukemia. Letters to the Editor. Farm Hosp. 2013;37(5):424-429.

31. European Society for Medical Oncology. Chronic myeloid leukaemia: ESMO Clinical Practice Guidelines for diagnosis, treatment and follow-up. Annals of Oncology. 2012; 23 (Suppl. 7).

32. Eiring E. Advanes in the treatment of chronic myeloid leukaemia. BMC Medicine. [Internet 2011[cited January 2015];9. Available from: http://www.biomedcentral.com/1741-7015/9/99

33. O Hare. Targeting the BCR-ABL signalling pathway in therapy

resistant philadelpia chromosome-positive leukaemia. Clin Cancer Res. 2011 January 15;17(2).

34. Talpaz M, et al. Phase I trial of AP24534 in patients with refractory chronic myeloid leukaemia (CML) and haematologic malignancies. J Clin Oncol. [Internet] 2010[cited January 2015]; 28. Available from: http://meetinglibrary.asco.org/content/53232-74

35. Hutter J. Childhood Leukemia. Pediatr Rev. 2010; 31:234-241.

36. Vormoor J, Chintagumpala M. Leukaemia and cancer in neonates. Semin Fetal Neonatal Med. 2012 Aug; 17(4):183-4.

37. Bresters D, Reus AC, Veerman AJ, van Wering ER, van der Does-van den Berg A, Kaspers GJ. Congenital leukaemia: the Dutch experience and review of the literature. Br J Haematol. [Internet] 2002[cited January 2015];117. Available from: http://www.ncbi.nlm.nih.gov/pubmed/12028017.

38. Krivtsov AV, Feng Z, Lemieux ME, Faber J, Vempati S, Sinha AU, et al. H3K79 methylation profiles define murine and human MLL-AF4 leukemias. Cancer Cell. [Internet] 2008[cited January 2015]; 14. Available from: http://www.ncbi.nlm.nih.gov/pubmed/18977325.

39. Zweidler-McKay PA, Hilden JM. The ABCs of Infant Leukemia. Curr Probl Pediatr Adolesc Health Care. [Internet] 2008[cited January 2015];38. Available from: http://www.ncbi.nlm.nih.gov/pubmed/18279790.

40. Van der Linden MH, Creemers S, Pieters R. Diagnosis and management of neonatal leukaemia. Seminars Fetal Neonatal Med. [Internet] 2012 [cited January 2015], 17. Available from: http://www.ncbi.nlm.nih.gov/pubmed/22510298

41. Creutzig U. Risk adapted treatment in Pediatric AML. 3rd

International Congress on Leukemia Lymphoma Myeloma. 2011 May 11-14 Istanbul, Turkey. Proceedings & Abstract Book. p. 210-2.

42. Creutzig U, Zimmermann M, Bourquin JP, Dworzak MN, Kremens B, Lehrnbecher T, et al. Favorable outcome in infants with AML after intensive first- and second-line treatment: an AML-BFM study group report. Leukemia [Internet]. 2012 Apr [cited January 2015]; 26(4). Available from: http://www.ncbi.nlm.nih.gov/pubmed/21968880

43. Roy A, Roberts I, Vyas P. Biology and management of transient abnormalmyelopoiesis (TAM) in children with Down syndrome. Seminars Fetal Neonatal Med. [Internet] 2012[cited January 2015]; 17. Available from: http://www.ncbi.nlm.nih.gov/pubmed/22421527

44. Xavier AC, Taub JW. Acute leukemia in children with Down syndrome. Haematol. [Internet] 2010[cited January 2015]; 95(7). Available from:http://www.haematologica.org/content/95/7/1043

45. Mitelman F, Johansson B and Mertens F. Mitelman Database of Chromosome Aberrations and Gene Fusions in Cancer [Internet]. Bethesda: NationalInstitutes of Health; 2013 [cited 2015 Jan 5]. Available from: http://cgap.nci.nih.gov/Chromosomes/Mitelman.

46. Ducasse K, Fernández JP, Salgado Carmen, et al. Characterization of febrile neutropenia episodes in children with acute myeloid leukemia and acute lymphoblastic leukemia. Rev Chilena Infectol [Internet]. 2014 [cited 2015 Jan 5]; 31 (3). Available from:http://www.scielo.cl/pdf/rci/v31n3/art13.pdf

47. Campbell M, Salgado C, Varas M. Clinical Guide 2010 Leukemia in persons under 15 years of age. Colombia: MINSAL; 2010. Available at:

http://web.minsal.cl/portal/url/item/7220fdc433e944a9e04001011f0113

b9.pdf

48. Salgado C, Becker A, Campbell M. National protocol for the treatment of acute myeloblastic leukemia. Colombia: MINSAL; 2006.

49. Gupta A, Singh M, Singh H. Infections in acute myeloid leukemia: an analysis of 382 febrile episodes. Med Oncol [Internet]. 2010 [cited January 2014]; 27. Available from: https://www.researchgate.net/publication/38012994_Infections_in_acut e_myel oid_leukemia_An_analysis_of_382_febrile_episodes

50. Gómez-Almaguer D, Flores-Jiménez JA, Cantú-Rodríguez O, Homero Gutiérrez-Aguirre C. Utility of hematopoietic cell transplantation in acute myeloid leukemia. Rev Hematol Mex [Internet]. 2012 [cited July 2013]; 13(2). Available from: http://www.medigraphic.com/pdfs/hematologia/re- 2012/re122f.pdf.

51. Ohtake S, Miyawaki S, Fujita H, Kiyoi H, Shinagawa K, Usui N, et al. Randomized study of induction therapy comparing standard-dose idarubicin with high-dose daunorubicin in adult patients with previously untreated acute myeloid leukemia: the JALSG AML201 Study. Blood [Internet]. 2011 [cited January 2014]; 117(8). Available at: http://www.ncbi.nlm.nih.gov/pubmed/20693429

52. Mulrooney DA, Yeazel MW, Kawashima T, et al. Cardiac outcomes in a cohort of adult survivors of childhood and adolescent cancer: retrospective analysis of the Childhood Cancer Survivor Study cohort. BMJ [Internet]. 2009 [cited January 2014]; 339. Available from http://www.bmj.com/content/339/bmj.b4606.

53. Whelan KStratton K, Kawashima T, Leisenring W, Hayashi S, Waterbor J, et al. Auditory complications in childhood cancer survivors: a report from the childhood cancer survivor study. Pediatr

Blood Cancer [Internet]. 2011 [cited Jan. 2014]; 57 (1). Available From http://www.ncbi.nlm.nih.gov/pubmed/21328523

54. Piñeros M, Pardo C, Otero J, Suárez A, Vizcaíno M, García S, et al. Protocol for surveillance and control of pediatric acute leukemias; 2010. [accessed January 2014]. Available en: http://190.27.195.165:8080/index.php?idcategoria=39005#

55. Llimpe Y, Monteza R, Ticlahuanca J, Rubio P. Acute myeloid leukemia subtype m2 with t(8;21) translocation variant and aml1/eto expression. Rev Peru Med Exp Salud Publica [Internet]. 2013 [cited January 2014]; 30(1). Available from: http://www.scielosp.org/scielo.php?script=sci_pdf&pid=S1726-46342013000100029&lng=en&nrm=iso&tlng=en.

56. Hernández Cruz C, Núñez Quintana A, Rodríguez Fraga Y. First case of acute myeloid leukemia treated in Cuba with high doses of anthracyclines in induction. Rev Cub Med [Internet]. 2012 [cited January 2014]; 51(2). Disponible en: http://scielo.sld.cu/scielo.php?script=sci_pdf&pid=S0034-75232012000200011&lng=es&nrm=iso&tlng=es

57. Fernandez HF, Rowe JM. Induction therapy in acute myeloid leukemia: intensifying and targeting the approach. Cur Op Hematol [Internet]. 2010 [cited January 2014]; 17(2). Available from: http://www.ncbi.nlm.nih.gov/pubmed/20087177

58. Pérez C, Agustí MA, Tornos P. Late anthracycline-induced cardiotoxicity. Med Clin (Barc) [Internet]. 2011 [cited 2 0 1 4 Jan 20];
133(8). Available at: http://www.elsevier.es/es-revista-medicina-clinica-2- articulo-cardiotoxicity-anthracycline-induced-ardia-

13140244.

59. Kolitz JE, George SL, Dodge RK. Dose escalation studies of cytarabine, daunorubicin, and etoposide with and without multidrug resistance modulation with PSC-833 in untreated adults with acute myeloid leukemia younger than 60 years: final induction results of Cancer and Leukemia Group B Study 9621. J Clin Oncol [Internet]. 2004 [cited June 2013]; 22(1). Available from:http://www.ncbi.nlm.nih.gov/pubmed/15514371

60. Fernandez HF, Sun Z, Yao X, Litzow MR, Luger SM, PaiettaEM, et al. Anthracycline dose intensification in acute myeloid leukemia. N Engl J Med [Internet]. 2011 [cited June 2015]; 361(13). Available from:http://www.nejm.org/doi/full/10.1056/NEJMoa0904544

61. Villela L, Bolaños-Meade J. Acute myeloid leukaemia: optimal management and recent developments. Drugs [Internet]. 2011 [cited June 2015]; 71(12). Available from:http://www.ncbi.nlm.nih.gov/pubmed/21861539

62. Menéndez Veitía A, González Otero A, Svarch Eva. Treatment o f acute myeloid leukemia in children in Cuba. Rev Cubana Hematol Inmunol Hemoter. [Internet]. 2013 [cited June from 2015]; 29(2). Available from:http://scielo.sld.cu/scielo.php?script=sci_arttext&pid=S0864-02892013000200010&lang=pt.

63. Puig H, Carroll WL, Meshinchi S, Arceci RJ. Biology, risk stratification, and therapy of pediatric acute leukemias: an update. J Clin Oncol [Internet]. 2011 [cited July 2013]; 29(5). Available from: http://www.ncbi.nlm.nih.gov/pubmed/21220611

64. Rubinitz JE. How I treat pediatric acute myeloid leukemia. Blood

[Internet]. 2012 [cited July 2013]; 119(25). Available from: http://www.ncbi.nlm.nih.gov/pubmed/22566607

65. Gibson B. The place of stem cell transplantation in 1st remission in Pediatric AML. 3rd International Congress on Leukemia Lymphoma Myeloma. 2011 May 11-14 Istanbul, Turkey. Proceedings & Abstract Book. p 200-3.

66. Gupta V, Tallman MS, Weisdorf DJ. Allogeneic hematopoietic cell transplantation for adults with acute myeloid leukemia: myths, controversies, and unknowns. Blood [Internet]. 2011 [cited July 2013]; 117(8). Available from: http://www.ncbi.nlm.nih.gov/pubmed/21098397

67. Vellenga E, van Putten W, Ossenkoppele GJ, Verdonck LF, Theobald M, Cornelissen JJ, et al. Autologous peripheral blood stem cell transplantation for acute myeloid leukemia. Blood [Internet]. 2011 [cited July 2013]; 118(23). Available from: http://www.ncbi.nlm.nih.gov/pubmed/21951683

68. De Witte T, Hagemeijer A, Suciu S, Belhabri A, Delforge M, Kobbe G, et al. Value of allogeneic versus autologous stem cell transplantation and chemotherapy in patients with myelodysplastic syndromes and secondary acute myeloid leukemia. Final results of a prospective randomized European Intergroup Trial. Haematologica [Internet]. 2010 [cited July 2013]; 95(10). Available from: http://www.ncbi.nlm.nih.gov/pubmed/20494931

69. Vardiman JW, Thiele J, Arber DA, Brunning RD, Borowitz MJ, Porwit A, et al. The 2008 revision of the World Health Organization (WHO) classification of myeloid neoplasms and acute leukemia: rationale and important changes. Blood [Internet]. 2009 [cited July 2013]; 114(5). Available from: http://www.ncbi.nlm.nih.gov/pubmed/19357394

70. Naoe T, Niederwieser D, Ossenkoppele GJ, Sanz MA, Sierra J, Burnett MS, et al. Diagnosis and management of acute myeloid leukemia in adults: recommendations from an international expert panel, on behalf of the European Leukemia Net. Blood [Internet]. 2010[cited July 2013]; 115(3). Available from: http://www.bloodjournal.org/content/bloodjournal/115/3/453.full.pdf? sso- checked=true

71. Paganini H, Santolaya M E. Diagnosis and treatment of febrile neutropenia in children with cancer. Consensus of the Latin American Society of Pediatric Infectious Diseases. Rev Chil Infectol [Internet]. 2011[cited July 2013]; 28(11). Available At: http://www.scielo.cl/scielo.php?pid=S0716-10182011000400003&script=sci_arttext

72. Villarroel M, Aviles C, Silva P, Guzmán A M, Poggi H, Alvarez A M, et al. Risk factor associated with invasive fungal disease in children with cancer and febrile neutropenia. A prospective multicenter evaluation. Pediatr Infect Dis J [Internet]. 2010 [cited July 2013]; 29(9). Available from: http://www.ncbi.nlm.nih.gov/pubmed/20616763

73. Dvorak C, Fisher B, Sung L. Antifungal prophylaxis in pediatric Hematology/Oncology: new choices & new data. Pediatr Blood Cancer [Internet]. 2012 [cited July 2013]; 59(1). Available from: http://www.ncbi.nlm.nih.gov/pubmed/22102607

74. Cavagnaro SF. Tumor lysis syndrome in Pediatrics. Rev Chil Pediatr [Internet]. 2011 [cited July 2013]; 82 (4): [approx. 6p.]. Available from: http://www.scielo.cl/scielo.php?pid=S0370-41062011000400009&script=sci_arttext.

75. Abu-Alfa A, Younes A. Tumor lysis syndrome and acute kidney injury: evaluation, preservation, and management. Am J Kidney Dis

[Internet]. 2011[cited July 2013]; 55 (S3). Available from: http://www.ncbi.nlm.nih.gov/pubmed/20420966

76. D'Orazio J: The tumor lysis syndrome: an oncological and metabolic emergency. In: Kiessling S, Goebel J, and Somers M, ed. Pediatric Nephrology in the ICU. Berlin-Heidelberg: Springer-Verlag; 2009.p. 201-18.

77. Zonfrillo M. Management of pediatric tumor lysis syndrome in the emergency department. Emerg Med Clin N Am [Internet]. 2011 [cited July 2013];

27(3). Available at: https://www.clinicalkey.es/#!/content/playContent/1- s2.0-S0733862709000376?returnurl=http:%2F%2Flinkinghub.elsevier.com %2Fretri eve%2Fpii%2FS0733862709000376%3Fshowall%3Dtrue&referrer=ht tp:%2F %2Fwww.ncbi.nlm.nih.gov%2Fpubmed%2F19646650

78. Moreno LP, Londoño D. Hyperleukocytosis associated with pulmonary and cerebral leukostasis in acute myeloid leukemia. Acta Med Coloma [Internet]. 2011 [cited July 2013]; 36: [approx. 2 p.]. Available en: http://www.scielo.org.co/scielo.php?script=sci_pdf&pid=S0120-24482011000200007&lng=en&nrm=iso&tlng=es

79. Tang JY, Gu LJ. Report on induction efficacy of protocol ALL-2005 and middle term follow-up of 158 cases of childhood acute lymphoblastic leukemia. ZhonghuaXue Ye XueZaZhi [Internet]. 2009; 30 (5). Available at: http://www.ncbi.nlm.nih.gov/pubmed/19799121

80. Kim H, Lee JH, Choi SJ, Lee JH, Seol M, Lee YS, et al. Risk score

model for fatal intracranial hemorrhage in acute leukemia. Leukemia [Internet]. 2006;

20(5). Available at: http://www.ncbi.nlm.nih.gov/pubmed/16525500

81. Ponce-Torres E, Ruíz-Rodríguez M del S, Alejo- González F, Hernández- Sierra JF, Pozos-Guillén Ade J. Oral manifestations in pediatric patients receiving chemotherapy for acute lymphoblastic leukemia. J Clin Pediatr Dent [Internet]. 2010; 34(3).   Available   at: http://www.ncbi.nlm.nih.gov/pubmed/20578668

82. Colombo A, Cipolla C, Beggiato M, Cardinale D. Cardiac toxicity of anticancer agents. Curr Cardiol Rep [Internet]. 2013 [cited February 2014];   15   (5).   Available   from: http://www.ncbi.nlm.nih.gov/pubmed/23512625

83. Kucharska W, Negrusz-Kawecka M, Gromkowska M. Cardiotoxicity of oncological treatment in children. Adv Clin Exp Med [Internet]. 2012 [cited February 2014]; 21(3). Available from: http://www.ncbi.nlm.nih.gov/pubmed/23214190

84. Eschenhagen T, Force T, Ewer MS, de Keulenaer GW, Suter TM, Anker SD, et al. Cardiovascular side effects of cancer therapies: a position statement from the Heart Failure Association of the European Society of Cardiology. Eur J Heart Fail [Internet]. 2011 [cited February 2014]; 13(1). Available from: http://www.ncbi.nlm.nih.gov/pubmed/21169385

85. Curado MP, Pontes T, Guerra-Yi ME, Cancela MC. Leukemia mortality trends among children, adolescents, and young adults in Latin America. Rev Panam Salud Pública [Internet]. 2011 [cited February   2014];29(2):   Available   from: http://www.ncbi.nlm.nih.gov/pubmed/21437366

86. Inaba H, Fan Y, Pounds S. Clinical and biologic features and treatment outcome of children with newly diagnosed acute myeloid

leukemia and hyperleukocytosis. Cancer [Internet]. 2008 [cited February 2014]; 113 (3). Available from: http://www.ncbi.nlm.nih.gov/pubmed/18484648

TABLES AND GRAPHS

Pediatric patients with acute myeloid leukemia according to age and sex.

Age (years)	Male		Female		Total	
	No	%	No	%	No	%
< 1	1	4.17	2	8.33	3	12.50
1 a 4	3	12.50	3	12.50	6	25.00
5 a 9	5	20.83	1	4.17	6	25.00
10 a 14	2	8.33	4	16.67	6	25.00
15 a 19	1	4.17	2	8.33	3	12.50
Total	12	50.00	12	50.00	24	100

Source: Medical records $X^2 = 4.000$p $= 0.406$

Pediatric patients with acute myeloid leukemia according to place of residence.

Residence	No	%
SanctiSpiritus	10	41.67
Villa Clara	6	25.00
Ciego de Avila	3	12.50
Cienfuegos	3	12.50
Granma	1	4.17
Matanzas	1	4.17
Total	24	100

Source: Medical records

Pediatric patients with acute myeloid leukemia according to skin color.

Skin color	No	%
White	21	87.5
Non-white	3	12.5
Total	24	100

Source: Medical records

Pediatric patients with acute myeloid leukemia according to nutritional status.

State nutritional	No	%
Delgado	2	8.33
Normopeso	18	75.00
Overweight	1	4.17
Obese	3	12.50
Total	24	100

Source: Medical records

Pediatric patients with acute myeloid leukemia according to nutritional status.

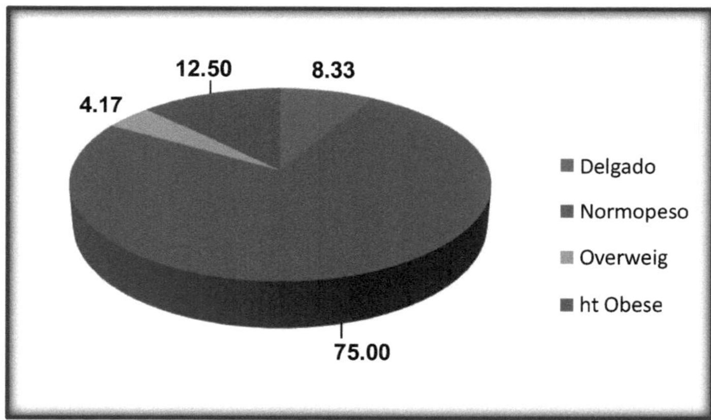

Source: Table 4

Pediatric patients with acute myeloid leukemia according to results at diagnosis.

Laboratory		No	%
Hemoglobin	< 11 gr/dl	23	95.83
	11 to 15 gr/dl	1	4.17
Leukocytes	< 5*10 /L^9	4	16.70
	5 to 11 *10 /L^9	2	8.30
	> 11*10 /L^9	18	75.00
Platelets	< 150*10 /L^9	17	70.80
	from 150 to 450 *10 /L^9	7	29.20

Source: Medical records

Table 6. Complications in pediatric patients with acute myeloid leukemia according to sex.

Complications	Sex						X^2	
	Male (n = 12)		Female (n = 12)		Total (n = 24)			
	No	%	No	%	No	%		
Sepsis	11	91.67	11	91.67	22	91.67	0.545	0.460
Febrile neutropenia	11	91.67	10	83.33	21	87.50	0.000	1.000
Hemorrhage before	9	75.00	6	50.00	15	62.50	1.623	0.202
Syndrome of	3	25.00	7	58.33	10	41.67	1.542	0.214
Bleeding during	5	41.67	1	8.33	6	25.00	2.000	0.157
Cardiotoxicity	4	33.33	4	33.33	8	33.33	0.000	1.000
Hyperleukocytosis	2	16.67	0	0.00	2	8.33	---	---

Source: Medical records

Complications in pediatric patients with acute myeloid leukemia according to sex.

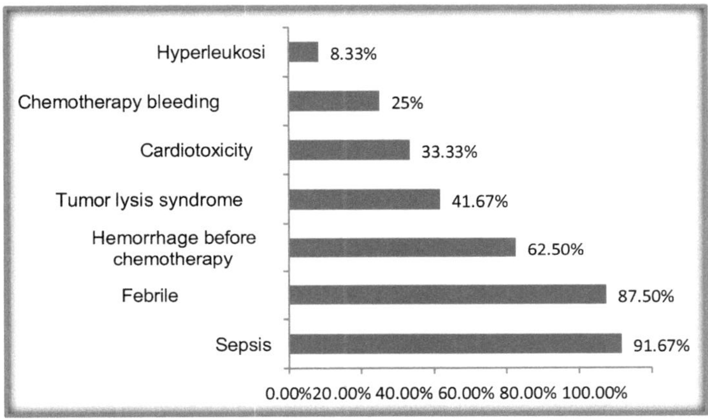

Source: Table 6

Table 7. Complications in pediatric patients with acute myeloid leukemia according to age.

Complications	< 1 year (n = 3)		1 a 4 (n = 6)		5 a 9 (n = 6)		10 a 14 (n = 6)		15 a 19 (n = 3)		X2	p
	No	%	No	%	No	%	No	%	No	%		
Sepsis	3	100	6	100	5	83.33	6	100	2	66.67	4.364	0.359
Febrile neutropenia	2	66.67	5	83.33	6	100	6	100	2	66.67	4.191	0.381
Hemorrhage before chemotherapy	2	66.67	3	50	4	66.67	5	83.33	1	33.33	2.667	0.615
Syndrome of lisistumoral	2	66.67	3	50	1	16.67	3	50.00	1	33.33	2.921	0.571
Hemorrhage during chemotherapy	0	0.00	3	50	2	33.33	0	0.00	1	33.33	5.333	0.255
Cardiotoxicity	1	33.33	4	66.67	1	16.67	2	33.33	0	0.00	5.250	0.263
Hyperleukosis	0	0	2	33.33	0	0	0	0	0	0	----	----

Source: Medical records

Table 8. Complications in pediatric patients with acute myeloid leukemia according to nutritional status.

Complications	Nutritional status								X2	p
	Delgado (n = 2)		Normopeso (n = 18)		Overweight (n = 1)		Obese (n = 3)			
	No	%	No	%	No	%	No	%		
Sepsis	1	50	17	94.44	1	100	3	100	5.091	0.165
Febrile neutropenia	1	50	16	88.89	1	100	3	100	3.175	0.366
Bleeding before chemotherapy	1	50	10	55.56	1	100	3	100	2.904	0.407
Syndrome of lisistumoral	0	0.00	8	44.44	0	0.00	2	66.67	2.971	0.396
Cardiotoxicity	0	0.00	4	22.22	1	100	3	100	10.000	0.019
Hemorrhage during chemotherapy	0	0.00	4	22.22	0	0.00	2	66.67	3.852	0.278
Hyperleukosis	0	0.00	0	0.00	0	0.00	2	66.67	15.273	0.002

Source: Medical records.

Table 9. Causes of death in the remission induction stage according to sex in pediatric patients with acute myeloid leukemia.

Causes of death in induction	Male (n = 12)		Female (n = 12)		Total (n = 24)	
	No	%	No	%	No	%
Severe sepsis	0	0.00	3	25.00	3	12.50
Intraparenchymal hemorrhage +CID	0	0.00	1	8.33	1	4.17
Intraparenchymal hemorrhage +SDMO	0	0.00	1	8.33	1	4.17
Intraparenchymal hemorrhage	1	8.33	1	8.33	2	8.33
Total	1	8.33	6	50.00	7	29.17

Source: Medical records $X^2 = 5.0420$ p $= 0.0247$

Current status of pediatric patients with acute myeloid leukemia.

Current status	No	%
Vivo	11	45.83
Died in induction	7	29.17
Deceased from another cause	6	25.00
Total	24	100

Source: Medical records.